INTO EVERYTHING

Magnesium is involved in almost every bodily function, participating in more than 50 biochemical reactions. It is vital to wound healing, growth, immune system function, temperature regulation, brain and nerve activity, muscle (including heart) action and the production of our basic energy source. Dr. Gaby explores the fascinating story of how magnesium works in our bodies—and how it can be used to foster health and fight many disease conditions, from heart problems to PMS.

ABOUT THE AUTHOR

Alan R. Gaby, M.D. has written many books and articles on the intimate connection between health and nutrition, including *B6: The Natural Healer* and *Preventing and Reversing Osteoporosis,* and speaks extensively on the topic. Dr. Gaby practices in Baltimore, Maryland.

MAGNESIUM

HOW AN IMPORTANT MINERAL HELPS PREVENT HEART ATTACKS AND RELIEVE STRESS

Alan R. Gaby, M.D.

Keats Publishing, Inc. New Canaan, Connecticut

Magnesium is not intended as medical advice. Its intent is solely informational and educational. Please consult a health professional should the need for one be indicated.

ISBN: 0-87983-602-4

Printed in the United States of America

Good Health Guides are published by
Keats Publishing, Inc.
27 Pine Street (Box 876)
New Canaan, Connecticut 06840-0876

Contents

THE IMPORTANCE OF MAGNESIUM

Magnesium deficiency is one of the most common nutritional problems in the industrialized world today. And because this mineral plays a key role in many basic biochemical processes, magnesium deficiency can result in a wide range of seemingly unrelated symptoms and medical conditions. Hardly a patient leaves my office without receiving a recommendation to take a magnesium supplement.

After decades of ignoring magnesium, the medical profession is finally beginning to recognize that some heart patients need magnesium supplements. However, the average doctor is still unaware of just how powerful magnesium can be as a cardiac "medication." Furthermore, most physicians do not know that magnesium is often effective against fatigue, diabetes, hypoglycemia, high blood pressure, asthma, muscle spasms, and fibromyalgia (a painful muscle disorder), or that this mineral can help prevent kidney stones, osteoporosis, and migraine headaches.

In thirteen years of practicing nutritional medicine, I have learned that nutrients work in the body as a team. No single vitamin or mineral can cure all of the problems that plague us. Nevertheless, magnesium so often makes a difference in our lives that it deserves special attention.

As we struggle to come to terms with a health care system that is too expensive and too often dangerous, it is reassuring to remember that we have reliable alternatives. In contrast to some prescription drugs that cost two dollars or more per day, magnesium supplements are generally under eight cents per day. In addition, while many prescription medicines can cause toxic side effects, magnesium is in general extremely safe. For millions of Americans, correcting magnesium deficiency could be one of the most important steps on the road back to health.

FUNCTIONS OF MAGNESIUM

Magnesium participates in more than 50 different biochemical reactions in the body. This mineral is necessary for growth and development, wound healing, immune system function, temperature regulation, and many activities of the brain and nervous system. Magnesium also plays a role in muscle contraction (both heart and skeletal muscle), muscle relaxation (i.e., reducing muscle spasm), and in regulating blood clotting. In addition, magnesium is required for the production of adenosine triphosphate (ATP), the molecular "power cell" on which the body depends to perform nearly all of its physical, mental, and biochemical work. As a result, magnesium is involved in some way or other in just about every bodily function.

WHY AN EPIDEMIC OF MAGNESIUM DEFICIENCY?

Considering the long list of conditions that can be prevented or treated with magnesium, a case can be made that there is an epidemic of magnesium deficiency in our society. There are three likely reasons why this is so: diet, stress, and drug interactions.

First, there is probably a lot less magnesium in the American diet than there was a century ago. Modern food processing and refining techniques cause considerable amounts of this mineral to be lost. For example, when whole wheat is refined to produce white flour, 85 percent of the magnesium is removed.[1] Refined sugar, which comprises about 19 percent of the calories in a typical American diet, has been almost completely stripped of the magnesium that occurs naturally in sugarcane.

These losses of magnesium are made even worse by farming techniques that deplete the soil of essential minerals. Traditional methods of farming include using manure and compost to increase the mineral content of the soil. In modern times, however, with the emphasis on producing higher crop yields, farmers use large amounts of inorganic fertilizers, which are often low in magnesium. For example, the overuse of nitrates, phosphates, and potassium salts as fertilizers, drains the soil of magnesium. In addition, the use of ammonia as a fertilizer causes magnesium to be leached from the soil.[2]

Many scientists and nutritionists do not understand that the quality of the soil directly affects the mineral content of foods. Indeed, nutrition textbooks often state that mineral-deficient soil will lower crop yield, but will not reduce the nutritional quality of crops that do grow. However, the facts indicate otherwise. The presence of a "goiter belt" in the midwestern United States proves that foods grown on iodine-deficient soil do not contain enough iodine to meet our requirements. The relationship between mineral concentrations in soil and food is also underscored by epidemics of selenium deficiency that occur in cattle that graze in low-selenium pastures. In the case of magnesium, dairy cattle and horses are sometimes stricken by a condition known as grass staggers, characterized by an unsteady gait, twitching, and muscle spasms. This disorder can be cured either by supplementing the diet with magnesium or by adding magnesium to the soil.[3]

Thus, our modern food supply starts off short in magnesium and, after the food processors are finished, the shortage is even worse. The typical American diet is, therefore, frequently low in magnesium. Dietary surveys have shown that many individuals fail to obtain the Recommended Dietary Allowance (RDA) of 350 mg per day. Magnesium has been found to be particularly low among adolescent girls, adult women, and elderly men, 75 to 85 percent of whom consume diets that provide less than the RDA.[4] In another study, the average magnesium intake of a group of high school and college women was only 36 percent of the RDA.[5] Even among a group of physically active United States Navy trainees (who presumably have ravenous appetites) 34 percent failed to meet the RDA for magnesium.[6]

MODERN LIVING INCREASES MAGNESIUM REQUIREMENTS

POLLUTION

The second likely reason that magnesium deficiency has become an epidemic is that the biochemical and emotional stresses of modern living cause us to lose more and, therefore, to need more of this important mineral. We live in an age in which we are bombarded by tens of thousands of chemical pollutants. It would be surprising if some of them did not interfere with the absorption or utilization of essential nutrients. In my book *B6: The Natural Healer*, I pointed out that a group of chemicals called hydrazines and hydrazides that are used in industry and agriculture and show up in our food supply are known to interfere with the effects of vitamin B6 in the body. The proliferation of these chemicals in our environment may explain why some of us need large doses of vitamin B6 to treat asthma, premenstrual syndrome, carpal tunnel syndrome, and other common problems.[7]

It is probable that chemical pollutants affect our magnesium requirements, as well. Aluminum, for example, is known to compete effectively for magnesium-binding sites in the body. The presence of even small amounts of aluminum might, therefore, block some of the normal biochemical functions of magnesium.[8] That possibility has important implications, given our widespread exposure to aluminum. This toxic metal is used to wrap foods and is the most commonly used metal in soft drink and beer cans. It is present as an additive in many foods and is added to some municipal water supplies to remove particulate matter. Aluminum is also a major ingredient in many antacids. Acid rain dissolves aluminum from the bedrock, resulting in very high aluminum concentrations in the groundwater in some areas of the country. This continual bombardment of our bodies with absorbable aluminum could have a significant impact on our magnesium status.

Lead, another ubiquitous toxin, also interacts with magnesium[9,10] and may, therefore, increase our magnesium requirements. Other pollutants may also reduce our magnesium status, although not much research has been done in that area.

STRESS

In addition to the biochemical stress caused by pollutants, we live in a world that engenders a great deal of emotional stress. Traffic jams, dysfunctional relationships, demanding jobs, financial worries, hyperactive children, and many other factors can add significant tension to our lives. Noise (from traffic, electrical appliances, fluorescent lights, and so on) is another significant, though sometimes forgotten, cause of stress in modern society.

The body responds to various types of stress by releasing epinephrine (adrenaline) and cortisol (a cortisonelike substance). Both of these compounds can cause magnesium to be released from cells and excreted in the urine.[11,12] Studies in both humans and animals have shown that exposure to noise or other types of stress will increase urinary magnesium excretion and reduce the magnesium in various tissues in the body.[13] Interestingly, individuals with a type A personality who are known to be especially susceptible to the damaging effects of stress are also more likely to experience stress-induced magnesium loss. Among a group of student-volunteers exposed to stress, 80 percent of type A students lost magnesium from their bodies, compared to only 44 percent of type B individuals.[14]

Thus, the combined effects of a magnesium-deficient diet, environmental pollution, and unprecedented mental stress most likely contribute to widespread magnesium deficiency.

DRUGS DEPLETE MAGNESIUM

Certain drugs have also been found to cause magnesium deficiency. These include thiazide diuretics (hydrochlorothiazide, chlorthalidone, etc.); loop diuretics (furosemide and bumetanide); some antibiotics (including gentamicin, carbenicillin, and amphotericin B); chemotherapeutic drugs (cis-platinum, vinblastine, and bleomycin); cyclosporine (used to prevent organ rejection in transplant patients); cortisone and related drugs; digoxin; and some of the stimulant drugs used to treat asthma. Chronic laxative abuse and excessive consumption of alcohol may also deplete magnesium.

DEFICIENCY AND DISEASE: A VICIOUS CYCLE

As you will see, magnesium deficiency can cause a number of different problems and may contribute to the development of certain chronic diseases. The situation is compounded, however, by a vicious cycle, in which illness aggravates magnesium deficiency, which, in turn, makes the illness even worse. To use the example mentioned previously, magnesium deficiency increases sensitivity to noise and causes a greater release of epinephrine in response to stress.[15] The additional amount of epinephrine in turn causes more magnesium to be lost. These factors would presumably set up a vicious cycle of greater magnesium depletion and more severe illness.

As disease progresses, cells lose their ability to function properly. Most of the cells of the body maintain a very high magnesium concentration relative to that in the blood serum. For example, there is about ten times as much magnesium inside the cells of a healthy heart as there is in the serum. This high intracellular concentration of magnesium is necessary for cells to perform their various biochemical tasks. However, maintaining this steep concentration gradient between cells and blood requires a great deal of energy. The laws of random motion cause magnesium ions to leak continually out of the cells and into the bloodstream. Each time a magnesium ion leaks out, another one must be pulled back in by special pumps that reside on the cell membrane. Pulling against a concentration gradient is analogous to swimming upstream or to carrying bowling balls up a hill, only to see them roll right back down. As inefficient as that sounds, that is how the body works. Indeed, a substantial proportion of the calories you burn each day are used to maintain higher concentrations of some nutrients inside cells than in the bloodstream.

When you become ill, some of the cells in your body may become less efficient at holding on to magnesium. The cell membrane may break down, allowing more magnesium to leak out. In addition, the cell membrane pumps that pull magnesium back in may also be weakened by disease. The end result is that disease itself can be a cause of magnesium deficiency. Since magnesium deficiency may have been one of the original causes of the disease, a vicious cycle of greater deficiency and increasingly severe disease may result.

Symptoms of Magnesium Deficiency

The symptoms of magnesium deficiency include fatigue, depression, anxiety, irritability, fear, restlessness, insomnia, faintness, hyperventilation, muscle cramps and twitches, intestinal complaints, tightness in the chest, poor attention, confusion, and memory loss. Most of these symptoms have more than one cause, and some are also manifestations of neurosis or other psychological problems. However, when magnesium deficiency is involved, correcting the deficiency will relieve the symptoms. When magnesium deficiency is severe, it can result in abnormal gait, vertigo, and even convulsions.

MAGNESIUM AND YOUR HEALTH

Magnesium Therapy: Oral versus Injectable

Foods rich in magnesium include whole grains, nuts, seeds, green vegetables, and animal foods. Including these foods in your diet will help prevent magnesium deficiency. However, if you have chronic symptoms or are subjected to excessive amounts of stress, taking magnesium supplements may be advisable.

In some of the studies described later, magnesium was given orally, whereas in others it was administered by intravenous or intramuscular injection. In my experience, taking magnesium orally usually relieves the symptoms caused by magnesium deficiency. However, a substantial minority of patients with these symptoms fail to improve after taking oral magnesium for months or even years. In these cases, administering magnesium by injection is necessary to overcome their medical problems. These people are probably locked into the vicious cycle of deficiency and disease I described previously. While they may not have any problem absorbing magnesium from their intestinal tract, the tissues in their body that are ailing have probably become less efficient at pulling magnesium into the cells. For example, an individual with heart disease may have subnormal amounts of magnesium in the heart muscle, despite normal levels elsewhere in the body.[16] The diseased tissues cannot obtain the amounts of magnesium they need unless the magnesium concentration in the bloodstream is raised well above normal.

Taking magnesium orally does not increase the serum magnesium concentration by more than about 10 to 20 percent. If you try to improve on that by swallowing more magnesium, you will get diarrhea, but not a higher serum magnesium level. Giving magnesium by intravenous injection, on the other hand, can increase serum levels by as much as 200 percent or more. Intramuscular injections also raise serum levels, although not as much as intravenous treatment. Although magnesium levels remain elevated only for several hours after an injection, that is apparently long enough to give the ailing cells what they need. The situation is comparable to a flood plain that is protected from the river by levees, but which becomes flooded when the water level rises above the levee. Sometimes, a series of magnesium injections breaks the vicious cycle by helping the ailing tissues to heal. In those cases, oral supplementation will maintain the improvement without additional injections. In other cases, however, tissue damage has progressed so far that periodic magnesium injections are required for months or even years.

A nutrition-oriented health care practitioner can help determine whether oral or injectable magnesium is appropriate for you. What is most important is that all of the tissues in your body have an adequate supply of this important mineral. The many ways in which magnesium can relieve illness and promote better health are described in the following sections.

Cardiovascular (Heart and Blood Vessel) Disease

Cardiovascular disease is the leading cause of death in the United States and is responsible for more than $50 billion annually in medical costs and lost productivity. Atherosclerosis, a progressive narrowing of the arteries, results in impaired blood flow to various tissues in the body. Atherosclerosis of the coronary arteries may promote angina and could contribute to a heart attack. If the blockage is in the arteries of the legs, one may experience intermittent claudication, a condition in which pain develops in the legs after walking. Congestive heart failure may or may not be caused by atherosclerosis in the coronary arteries. In the case of cardiomyopathy, the heart muscle becomes diseased and heart failure occurs, despite adequate blood flow to the area.

Doctors prescribe a number of different types of medications to prevent and treat cardiovascular disease. Aspirin is used to reduce the tendency of blood platelets to form clots. Drugs known as calcium channel blockers are given to dilate narrowed arteries or to prevent them from going into spasm. Fibrinolytic drugs (commonly called clot busters) are administered at the first sign of a heart attack to reopen arteries that have been occluded by a blood clot. Another class of drugs known as angiotensin-converting enzyme (ACE) inhibitors is also used to dilate blood vessels.

It is noteworthy that magnesium can accomplish single-handedly many of the objectives that cardiologists try to achieve with these various drugs. Magnesium simultaneously inhibits platelet clumping, enhances fibrinolytic activity, blocks calcium channels, and promotes dilation of blood vessels. Magnesium also does something that none of these drugs can do: it improves the efficiency with which heart muscle cells function, thereby allowing an oxygen-deprived heart muscle to get by with less oxygen. That effect is particularly important, since optimizing cellular metabolism in times of cardiac stress may mean the difference between cell recovery and cell death.

The ability of magnesium to protect the heart from damage was demonstrated many years ago in a study by Nobel Prize winner Hans Selye, M.D.[17] Rats were subjected to surgical occlusion of the left coronary artery, which resulted in a restriction of blood flow to a portion of the heart. Among rats fed a standard laboratory diet that contained supposedly adequate amounts of magnesium, every one developed a myocardial infarction (heart attack). However, among those provided additional dietary magnesium for five days prior to occlusion of the artery, only 29 percent suffered an infarction. A more recent study performed at the George Washington University College of Medicine demonstrated that magnesium deficiency renders heart muscle more vulnerable to injury.[18]

Magnesium and Heart Attacks

It was reported more than 35 years ago that administering magnesium during a heart attack can save lives. In one study,[19] more than 100 patients with heart disease, at least one-third of whom had suffered an acute heart attack, were given intramuscular injections of magnesium sulfate (0.5 to 1.0 g every 5 days for 12 injections). Only one death occurred: a mortality rate of less than 1 percent. These results were a dramatic improvement over the previous year, when magnesium was not used. In that year, the death rate among 196 similar patients was 30 percent. Similar results were reported in a study in South Africa.[20]

Despite these rather impressive results, magnesium therapy for heart attacks did not catch on and no additional studies were performed for nearly 30 years. However, in 1986, the first of three studies was published that supported the earlier research. These recent studies were also more acceptable from a scientific standpoint, since they all used the double-blind methodology, where half of the patients received a placebo. Scientists prefer double-blind studies, because they can distinguish purely psychological benefits from those resulting from the treatment itself.

In the 1986 study from Denmark,[21] 273 patients with suspected acute myocardial infarction received either intravenous magnesium or a placebo. The infusions were started immediately on admission to the hospital and were continued for 48 hours. During the four weeks after treatment, there were 71 percent fewer deaths in patients given magnesium than in those who received the placebo. In addition, there were 24 percent fewer heart attacks in the magnesium group than in the placebo group. Evidently, administering magnesium in the early stages of a heart attack can help the injured heart muscle recover, rather than allowing it to progress to permanent damage. That possibility is supported by the results of the animal study by Selye described previously.

In 1990, an Israeli study published in the *American Journal of Cardiology*[22] confirmed the findings of the Danish researchers. One hundred three patients suffering heart attacks received a 48-hour intravenous infusion of magnesium or a placebo infusion. Of those in the magnesium group, only 2 percent died in the hospital, compared to 17 percent of those in the placebo group. Thus, magnesium reduced the death rate from heart attacks by an astounding 88 percent. In addition, as in the Danish study, magnesium therapy appeared to prevent some impending heart attacks from progressing to the real thing.

The most recent study, from England, was also the largest, enrolling 2,316 patients suspected of suffering a heart attack.[23] In that study, the four-week mortality rate was 24 percent lower in the magnesium group than in the placebo group. Although still statistically significant, the benefits of magnesium were not as great as in the studies mentioned previously. The difference in results may be due to the fact that patients in the British study received magnesium up to 24 hours after the onset of chest pain, whereas, in the Danish and Israeli studies, treatment was started within three to five hours after symptoms developed. It is well-known that any treatment for a heart attack becomes less effective, the longer one waits to administer it. Most scientists agree that, for best results, treatment should be started within six hours of the onset of chest pain. In addition, more than one-third of the patients in the British study received fibrinolytic drugs, which have also been shown to reduce heart attack deaths. Some of the benefits of magnesium may have therefore been masked by improvements due to the use of fibrinolytic drugs.

The currently accepted treatment for an acute heart attack includes fibrinolytic drugs (clot-busters), often combined with aspirin or heparin to thin the blood. However, the results of magnesium therapy, in terms of lives saved, are better than those of any of the treatments now in vogue. In addition, magnesium is safer. In contrast to fibrinolytic drugs which cause bleeding in the brain in one of every 170 or so patients, magnesium does not promote bleeding or any other serious side effects. Furthermore, in this era of runaway health care costs, the cost advantage of magnesium cannot be ignored. Whereas the fibrinolytic drugs TPA (tissue plasminogen activator) and streptokinase cost $2,300 and $280, respectively, per dose, a 48-hour infusion of magnesium costs less than five dollars.

Thus, for many reasons, magnesium should be considered the treatment of choice for most heart attack patients. A soon-to-be-completed study of 40,000 patients is comparing the effects of magnesium to those of fibrinolytic drugs and other treatments. Hopefully, this study will provide definitive information about what treatment or combination of treatments produces the greatest benefits with the least risk.

Arrhythmias

Cardiac arrhythmias (heart rhythm abnormalities) occur frequently in people with heart disease and in some who do not have heart disease. Certain arrhythmias are relatively benign, even though they may cause disturbing symptoms. Others are more serious and may even result in sudden death. Magnesium deficiency can cause a number of different abnormalities of heart rhythm. Magnesium has been used successfully to treat various arrhythmias, including premature ventricular contractions,[24] arrhythmias due to digitalis toxicity,[25] and a life-threatening arrhythmia known as *torsades de pointes*.[26] In the heart attack studies described earlier, some of the reduction in mortality associated with magnesium therapy was ascribed to a lower incidence of severe arrhythmias. Magnesium injections have also been found to reduce the number of arrhythmias occurring after cardiac surgery.[27]

Atherosclerosis

Atherosclerosis, also called hardening of the arteries, is a common problem among Americans. The progressive narrowing of arteries can contribute to the development of heart attacks, angina, intermittent claudication (to be discussed later in this section), ulcers on the feet or legs, and even gangrene. Although most doctors focus on dietary fat and cholesterol as the main causes of atherosclerosis, the condition is actually very complicated and most likely has numerous causes. Deficiencies of various vitamins and minerals, particularly vitamin B_6, vitamin C, vitamin E, folic acid, zinc, copper, chromium, and selenium, all promote the development of atherosclerosis.

Magnesium also appears to play a crucial role in atherosclerosis prevention. In one study, addition of cholesterol and cholic acid to the diet of rats caused both atherosclerosis and signs of magnesium deficiency, even though the amount of magnesium in the diet was usually adequate for rats. The development of atherosclerosis was prevented by increasing the amount of dietary magnesium fourfold.[28] In a similar study, rabbits fed a high-cholesterol diet developed atherosclerosis in the aorta. Although the amount of magnesium in this diet (400 mg per day) was enough to satisfy the usual requirement for rabbits, providing additional magnesium reduced the severity of atherosclerosis in the aorta.[29]

Effect on Serum Cholesterol

In these studies, magnesium prevented the development of atherosclerosis, even though it did not stop the rise in serum cholesterol produced by cholesterol feeding. Evidently, magnesium somehow protects the blood vessel wall from damage or minimizes the damage caused by cholesterol. However, other research has shown that magnesium does, indeed, improve cholesterol levels, an effect which would be expected to provide additional protection against atherosclerosis.

Cholesterol is found in the bloodstream in several different forms. Most are associated with an increased risk of developing heart disease. Reducing total serum cholesterol may, therefore, lower your risk. High-density lipoprotein (HDL) cholesterol, on the other hand, actually appears to reduce the risk of heart disease and has therefore been termed "good cholesterol." Doctors often attempt to lower total cholesterol levels while at the same time increasing HDL cholesterol concentrations. In one study, magnesium supplements accomplished both of those objectives. Sixteen patients with elevated total cholesterol and abnormally low HDL cholesterol levels received 400 mg of magnesium daily for an average of 118 days. The average total cholesterol level fell from 297 to 257 milligrams per deciliter, while HDL cholesterol increased from 35.2 to 46.7 mg/dl. Both of these changes were statistically significant and would be expected to reduce cardiovascular risk.[30] In another study, magnesium had no effect on total serum cholesterol; the effect on HDL cholesterol was not investigated.

Angina

The chest pain that often occurs in heart patients during exertion or stress is called angina. Many treatments have been tried for this common condition, but none are universally effective. In 1958, a South African physician reported that, in patients with angina, an appreciable number responded to magnesium injections, "sometimes in a dramatic and almost unbelievable manner, and this after all conventional and accepted methods of therapy had failed and sufferers had lost hope of ever obtaining relief."[31] These encouraging results were confirmed eleven years later in a report by a British doctor. Twenty-nine patients with angina were treated with magnesium injections. The usual dose was 1 to 2 g of magnesium sulfate given once a week for eight weeks. Fifteen of the 29 patients reported complete relief of symptoms. Seven of these patients remained symptom-free for more than two years. In general, intravenous injections were more effective than intramuscular injections.[32]

The frequency and severity of angina are sometimes affected by psychological factors, and placebo therapy can be surprisingly beneficial in some cases. Consequently, the effectiveness of magnesium against angina cannot be considered proven. Nevertheless, this treatment holds great promise and should be investigated further. In my medical practice, I have seen some patients respond to magnesium injections after other treatments had failed.

Intermittent Claudication

When atherosclerosis occurs in the legs, the resulting impairment of blood flow may cause a condition known as intermittent claudication. Individuals suffering from this problem have difficulty walking any great distance, because pain in their legs forces them to stop before they have gone very far. One physician reported in 1969 that magnesium injections produced marked improvement in 13 of 19 patients with intermittent claudication.[33]

In a more recent study, magnesium was also found to be effective when taken orally. Nineteen patients with intermittent claudication received 250 mg of magnesium hydroxide twice a day for 60 days. Prior to magnesium treatment, the patients were asked to walk on a treadmill until the pain in their legs forced them to stop. This treadmill test was repeated after 30 and 60 days of magnesium supplementation. The average walking distance increased by 51 percent after 30 days, and by 82 percent after 60 days. Twelve of the 19 patients were able to walk at least 50 percent longer than they could before taking magnesium. Although serum levels of magnesium were normal in these patients, the magnesium content of muscle was found to be low. However, muscle magnesium levels rose promptly after magnesium therapy was started. This study demonstrates that magnesium deficiency is common in individuals with intermittent claudication and suggests that magnesium supplementation allows most patients to increase their walking distance.[34] Because there was no placebo group in this study, the beneficial effect of magnesium against intermittent claudication cannot be considered proven.

Congestive Heart Failure and Cardiomyopathy

When the heart becomes weak, a number of changes occur which cause fluid to back up into the lungs. This condition, called congestive heart failure, can cause shortness of breath, weakness, and weight loss, and is the eventual cause of death in many heart patients. Congestive heart failure may result from impaired blood flow due to atherosclerosis or from primary disease of the heart muscle, called cardiomyopathy.

Autopsies performed on the hearts of individuals who died from congestive heart failure reveal changes similar to those seen in animals fed a magnesium-deficient diet.[35] That observation suggests that magnesium deficiency may play a role in the development of this condition. As I mentioned before, heart disease itself causes a loss of magnesium from heart muscle, which, in turn, further exacerbates the disease. In one study, patients with cardiomyopathy had 65 percent less magnesium in their heart muscle than did healthy individuals.[36]

Although no studies have been published on magnesium treatment of congestive heart failure, I have seen some rather remarkable results in a few patients. One patient was in the final stages of heart failure due to cardiomyopathy, having declined progressively over a number of years. At the time I was consulted, he had been in the hospital intensive care unit for a full month, being kept alive only by a continuous infusion of dobutamine, a powerful heart-stimulating drug. The doctors asked the patient's wife to make sure his affairs were in order, so that they could turn off the dobutamine drip and let him die. Instead, after consulting with me, she insisted that he be given a trial of magnesium therapy. Not wanting to deny the request of a dying patient's wife, the doctors started giving the patient 1 g of magnesium sulfate intramuscularly, once every four days. The patient improved rapidly and was sent home, where he continued to receive magnesium injections for two years until his death. During that time, if he went longer than four days without an injection, his condition would deteriorate, only to improve again after receiving more magnesium.

Hypertension

Hypertension (high blood pressure) is a common problem, affecting millions of Americans. Individuals with hypertension have an increased risk of developing a heart attack or stroke. Although there are many causes of hypertension, magnesium deficiency appears to be an important factor in some cases. In one study, individuals with hypertension had lower levels of magnesium in their red blood cells than people with normal blood pressure. Furthermore, the higher the blood pressure was, the lower were the magnesium levels.[37] Magnesium depletion is known to promote spasm in arteries, and chronic spasm will cause the blood pressure to rise. It is therefore important that people with hypertension have adequate levels of magnesium in their body. Unfortunately, some of the same factors that promote high blood pressure (such as emotional stress, noise, and ingestion of alcohol) also deplete the body of magnesium.

Magnesium supplements have been shown to lower blood pressure in some studies, although the results have not been consistent. In one experiment, administering 600 mg per day of magnesium to 21 individuals with hypertension resulted in a significant reduction in blood pressure.[38] In another study, 39 patients who were receiving diuretics (water pills) for hypertension or congestive heart failure were given either 365 mg per day of magnesium or no magnesium supplement at all. All of the patients were given potassium. This study was undertaken because most diuretics cause losses of magnesium and potassium in the urine and a deficiency of these minerals can raise the blood pressure. After six months of treatment, there was a significant drop in both systolic and diastolic blood pressure in the magnesium group. There was no significant decrease in blood pressure in those who did not receive magnesium.[39]

The results of this study may explain why the blood pressure-lowering effect of diuretics often diminishes with time. With continued treatment, more and more magnesium and potassium are lost, and that tends to push the blood pressure back up. Furthermore, there is evidence that diuretic-induced magnesium and potassium deficiency may be more dangerous than the high blood pressure for which the diuretic was prescribed. In the landmark Multiple Risk Factor Intervention Trial (MR FIT), certain groups of men with hypertension who received diuretics had a higher death rate than those whose hypertension was left untreated.[40] It has been suggested that some of these men died from heart rhythm disturbances (arrhythmias) caused by deficiency of one or both of these minerals. As a result, many physicians have abandoned mineral-depleting diuretics as a treatment for hypertension. If you must take a diuretic, it may be advisable for you to supplement with potassium and magnesium. However, not all diuretics deplete these minerals, and some actually cause the levels to rise. If you are taking a diuretic, do not self-treat with potassium and magnesium. Talk to your doctor about the advisability of taking supplements.

Some studies have found magnesium to be ineffective against hypertension.[41,42] Clearly, there are many different causes of this common problem, and no single therapy will be universally effective. However, because of its low cost, safety, and importance for the cardiovascular system in general, magnesium therapy should not be overlooked in people with hypertension.

Strokes

One of the most important risk factors for developing a stroke is hypertension, just discussed. To the extent that magnesium prevents hypertension, it would also reduce stroke risk. In addition, magnesium deficiency would increase the risk of the carotid arteries (in the neck) or the arteries in the brain going into spasm and choking off the blood supply to areas of the brain.[43] This impairment of blood flow could lead to a transient ischemic attack (TIA; prestroke) or a stroke. That possibility is more than academic, since stroke patients have been shown to have a deficiency of magnesium, both in the bloodstream and in the cerebrospinal fluid (the fluid that surrounds the brain).[44] Magnesium supplementation may therefore play an important role in the prevention of strokes.

Mitral Valve Prolapse

Mitral valve prolapse is a condition in which the leaflets of the mitral valve protrude into the left ventricle of the heart. It is caused by an abnormality of the connective tissue in the mitral valve. Approximately one in 20 people has a prolapsed mitral valve. Although this abnormality is considered relatively benign, rarely causing significant heart disease, individuals with mitral valve prolapse frequently suffer from chest pain, muscle cramps, shortness of breath, dizziness, cardiac arrhythmias, fatigue, palpitations, light-headedness, and anxiety. Doctors are usually unable to determine the cause of these symptoms, although they are similar to those of magnesium deficiency.

In a study of 24 individuals with mitral valve prolapse who had some combination of the symptoms just listed, red blood cell magnesium levels were below normal in two-thirds of the cases.[45] Magnesium deficiency is therefore a common finding in people with mitral valve prolapse, and may be responsible for some of the associated symptoms. To evaluate that possibility, 52 patients with mitral valve prolapse were given magnesium supplements orally for periods ranging from one month to four years. Muscular symptoms improved markedly and in some cases anxiety, fatigue, arrhythmias, and general sense of well-being also improved.[46] Other researchers have found similar results. In one study, individuals with mitral valve prolapse who took magnesium supplements had improvements in palpitations, chest pains, muscle cramps, and blood vessel spasms (Raynaud's phenomenon).[47]

It has been suggested that magnesium deficiency or a genetic abnormality of magnesium metabolism may cause the connective tissue of the mitral valve to develop abnormally, resulting in prolapse of the valve. In the studies described previously, magnesium supplementation did not correct the abnormal structure of the mitral valve, even though various symptoms improved. It is likely that, once the mitral valve has developed, the prolapse cannot be corrected. However, it is possible that assuring optimal magnesium intake prenatally and during the early years of life may prevent mitral valve prolapse from developing in the first place.

MAGNESIUM AND OTHER HEALTH PROBLEMS

Fatigue

Fatigue or tiredness is a common problem, affecting more than half of the people who visit the doctor. Although a thorough medical evaluation is important for anyone who suffers from persistent fatigue, too often no specific cause for the problem is found. Conventional medicine has little to offer most people who are tired, except to reassure them there is nothing seriously wrong with them.

Several decades ago, a French scientist named Laborit formulated the hypothesis that fatigue is sometimes caused by inefficient energy production within the cells. He theorized that fatigue might be relieved by enriching the cells with the nutrients that are involved in energy production. Potassium and magnesium, in the form of potassium magnesium aspartate, were considered ideal candidates for this purpose.

Laborit's hypothesis was first successfully tested in animals.[48] Subsequently, studies in humans suggested that potassium magnesium aspartate is also an effective treatment for fatigue in humans. Four uncontrolled studies and three double-blind studies were performed; all produced similar results. Between 75 and 91 percent of patients given 2 g per day (four 500 mg capsules) of potassium magnesium aspartate reported pronounced relief of fatigue. In contrast, only 5 to 25 percent of those receiving a placebo improved. A beneficial effect was usually noted after four to ten days.

In my experience, some patients are able to discontinue potassium magnesium aspartate after a few months without experiencing a recurrence of fatigue, whereas others must continue taking the supplement. It is important to note that some commercially available products are not true aspartates, but rather "aspartate complexes." The difference is how tightly the potassium and magnesium are bound to the aspartate. While I have had good success in my medical practice using true potassium magnesium aspartate, I do not know if the aspartate complexes work very well. True potassium magnesium aspartate contains 35 mg of magnesium and 99 mg of potassium in each 500-mg capsule.

Chronic Fatigue Syndrome

Magnesium may also be of value in the treatment of chronic fatigue syndrome (CFS). This condition, first described in the early 1980s, is believed to be caused by a virus, although abnormalities of the immune system may also be involved. CFS is more severe than the usual type of fatigue that people experience. Individuals with CFS are often so exhausted that they spend most of their time in bed and are unable to lead a normal life. There are many theories about the cause of CFS and many treatments have been tried, most without success.

Whatever the cause of CFS, magnesium therapy has the potential to relieve the symptoms. As mentioned earlier, chronic illness can cause magnesium depletion, which can, in turn, make the illness worse. This vicious cycle may be a factor in CFS. In one study, magnesium levels were significantly lower in the red blood cells of patients with CFS than in healthy individuals. Consequently, a double-blind study was performed to assess the value of magnesium injections. Thirty-two patients with CFS received either intramuscular magnesium sulfate (1 g weekly for 6 weeks) or placebo injections. Of the 15 patients given magnesium, 12 (80 percent) reported improvements in their energy level, emotional state, and degree of pain. In 7 of the 15 cases, fatigue was completely eliminated. In contrast, only 3 (18 percent) of the 17 placebo-treated patients improved, and in no case was fatigue completely eliminated. The difference between magnesium therapy and placebo was highly statistically significant.[49]

In other studies, no evidence of magnesium deficiency was found in individuals with CFS.[50,51] In one of these studies, a single intravenous magnesium injection failed to relieve fatigue. However, in my experience, a series of magnesium injections is often beneficial, even if the first treatment does not produce results. Since magnesium injections are safe and inexpensive, they are worth trying in patients with CFS. I have found that combining magnesium with calcium, B vitamins, and vitamin C is often more effective than using magnesium alone.[52]

Athletic Performance

In addition to being helpful for fatigue, magnesium supplements may also enhance athletic performance. In one double-blind study, 26 volunteers participated in a 7-week weight-training program. Each individual received either a placebo or a magnesium supplement. At the end of the weight-training program, those in the magnesium group had increased their strength significantly more than those in the placebo group.[53] In another study, 14 athletes were given a magnesium supplement and a placebo, during two different 4-week periods. Tests indicated that the magnesium supplement increased the efficiency of oxygen utilization, suggesting that magnesium may enhance aerobic fitness.[54] Thus, magnesium supplementation may improve both muscle strength and endurance in athletes.

Diabetes

More than 10 million Americans suffer from diabetes, a condition in which blood sugar levels are abnormally elevated. Longstanding diabetes is associated with a number of complications, including heart disease, atherosclerosis (hardening of the arteries), neuropathy (nerve damage), nephropathy (kidney disease), and retinopathy (damage to the retina of the eye). Diabetics can reduce their risk of developing these complications by taking measures to maintain their blood sugar level within or near the normal range. These include getting regular exercise; avoiding sugar, caffeine, and alcohol, while emphasizing high fiber complex carbohydrate foods; using nutritional supplements such as chromium, biotin, manganese, zinc, and copper;[55] and taking blood sugar-lowering medications when necessary.

Magnesium deficiency appears to be extremely common among diabetics. Several studies have shown that serum magnesium is lower in diabetics than in healthy individuals.[56,57,58] Magnesium levels in these studies were lowest in diabetics that had retinopathy. Diabetes may itself contribute to the development of magnesium deficiency. Chronic elevations of blood sugar would tend to upset the acid/base balance of the blood, causing magnesium to leak out of the cells and be excreted in the urine. This loss of magnesium then becomes part of a vicious cycle, since magnesium deficiency may actually make the diabetes worse.

In a group of 67 adult-onset diabetics, glucose tolerance was found to be directly related to the concentration of magnesium in the blood plasma. In other words, those with normal blood levels of magnesium were able to metabolize glucose more efficiently than those with lower magnesium levels.[59] Further research demonstrated that magnesium supplementation may in fact improve glucose tolerance. Twelve elderly individuals were given either a magnesium supplement or a placebo for four weeks. Elderly people were chosen for this study because they tend to have mildly impaired glucose tolerance and lower magnesium levels than young adults. Compared with the placebo, magnesium treatment significantly improved glucose handling.[60]

These studies demonstrate that magnesium deficiency is common in diabetics and that this deficiency may contribute both to the severity of the diabetes and to the risk of retinopathy. Cardiovascular disease, a common complication of diabetes, may also be caused in part by magnesium deficiency. The weight of evidence suggests that diabetics should receive magnesium supplements. However, self-medication can be dangerous in diabetics, particularly in those who have associated kidney disease or are taking blood sugar-lowering medication. If you have diabetes and wish to take magnesium or other nutritional supplements, you should consult a practitioner who is knowledgeable about nutrition.

Hypoglycemia

Hypoglycemia (also called reactive hypoglycemia) is a common condition in which the blood sugar falls to abnormally low levels. Symptoms of hypoglycemia include fatigue, anxiety, irritability, sweating, abdominal burning, headaches, insomnia, chest pain, and intense hunger. These symptoms are typically brought on by failure to eat frequently enough and are usually relieved by eating. Individuals with hypoglycemia often crave sugar, because eating something sweet rapidly relieves the symptoms. However, this "sugar high" soon ends in a "crash" and, over the long run, continually eating sweets usually makes the condition worse.

Although hypoglycemia is on rare occasions a sign of serious illness, most individuals with hypoglycemia do not have a significant medical problem. Some hypoglycemics eventually develop diabetes, but most do not. Nevertheless, the symptoms of hypoglycemia can be quite troublesome, and are sometimes severe enough to interfere with daily living.

The nutritional treatment of hypoglycemia is similar to that for diabetes. Avoiding refined sugar, caffeine, and alcohol; emphasizing high-fiber foods; and doing regular exercise are usually helpful. Eating between-meal snacks often prevents the blood sugar from falling too low before the next meal. Nutritional supplements such as chromium and the B vitamins are also helpful. In many cases, hypoglycemics benefit from small amounts of thyroid hormone or from supplements or medication that support the adrenal gland.

Magnesium also plays a significant role in preventing hypoglycemia. In one study, 22 individuals with reactive hypoglycemia (documented by glucose tolerance tests) received either 340 mg per day of magnesium or a placebo for 6 weeks. Some, though not all, of the people being studied had laboratory evidence of magnesium deficiency. Of those given magnesium, 57 percent reported feeling better, compared to only 25 percent of those taking the placebo. Three of the individuals in the study had glucose tolerance tests taken both before and after they received magnesium. In each case, the drop in blood sugar during the test was greatly reduced by magnesium.[61] This study shows that magnesium supplements may help prevent hypoglycemia and the symptoms associated with it.

Asthma

As many as 10 million Americans suffer from asthma, a condition in which the bronchial passages go into spasm and interfere with normal breathing. The incidence of asthma has increased and the death rate from asthma has nearly doubled in the United States during the past ten years. A deterioration of indoor and outdoor air pollution has most likely contributed to these bleak statistics. In addition, some experts blame part of the rise in the asthma death rate on the very medications used to treat asthma. Stimulant drugs such as theophylline, terbutaline, and metaproterenol can sometimes cause serious side effects, including high blood pressure and life-threatening heart rhythm disturbances (arrhythmias). It is probably no accident that these side effects are also manifestations of magnesium deficiency and that some asthma drugs have been shown to reduce blood levels of magnesium.[62,63]

Since magnesium promotes relaxation of bronchial muscles, its deficiency would increase the likelihood that the bronchi will go into spasm and cause an asthma attack. Magnesium deficiency can also increase the release of histamine into the bloodstream, thereby increasing allergic reactivity in general.[64] For both of these reasons, asthmatics should make sure to obtain an adequate supply of magnesium.

Asthma is frequently associated with magnesium deficiency. In one study, serum magnesium levels were below normal in half of 26 asthmatics during an acute attack and in 8 percent of 40 asthmatics who were not experiencing an acute attack.[65] The prevalence of magnesium deficiency may actually be much greater than those numbers suggest, since blood levels of magnesium do not fall below normal until total-body magnesium has become severely depleted.

It was shown as early as 1940 that acute asthma attacks, even severe ones, could be aborted by administering magnesium injections.[66] It was not until recently, however, that the medical community began to take a serious look at magnesium as a treatment for asthma. In one study, 10 patients with asthma received an intravenous infusion of magnesium. Wheezing and shortness of breath improved within two minutes and lung function tests provided objective confirmation of these improvements. The results of magnesium therapy were similar to those of albuterol inhalation, a standard emergency room treatment for asthma.[67]

These beneficial effects of magnesium were confirmed in another study conducted at the Emergency Department of the Medical College of Pennsylvania.[68] Thirty-eight patients with acute asthma attacks that had failed to respond to the usual emergency room treatments were given an intravenous infusion of magnesium sulfate (1.2g over a twenty-minute period) or a placebo infusion. Of those given the placebo, 79 percent required hospitalization, compared to only 37 percent of those given magnesium. This difference was statistically significant. One patient felt lightheaded during the magnesium infusion (intravenous magnesium sometimes causes a transient fall in blood pressure), but no other side effects occurred.

This study represents a major advance in the treatment of asthma. As many as 30 percent of patients with acute asthma attacks fail to respond to standard treatment and must therefore be hospitalized. Deaths from acute asthma are not uncommon and appear to be on the rise. Furthermore, some of the drugs used to treat asthma can cause serious or even life-threatening side effects. Magnesium is not only an effective alternative to these treatments, it is much safer, as well.

In my office over the past ten years, I have treated dozens of cases of acute asthma with intravenous magnesium, combined with calcium, vitamin C, and B vitamins. In nearly every case, the asthma improved markedly or subsided completely within thirty seconds to two minutes. In a small proportion of cases, a second injection was needed. I have found that using this combination of nutrients results in a more pronounced and long-lasting effect than giving magnesium alone. Because this nutrient injection works faster, lasts longer, has far fewer side effects, and costs less than conventional treatments, it should be seriously considered as the "treatment of choice" for acute asthma attacks.[69]

Although oral magnesium supplementation has not been well studied as a treatment or preventative for asthma, I always advise asthmatic patients to take extra magnesium. As mentioned earlier, asthma is often associated with magnesium deficiency, which may be aggravated by some of the drugs used to treat asthma. Taking extra magnesium may not only reduce the severity of asthma, but could decrease the risk of side effects from asthma medications.

Additional potassium may also be advisable if you are taking asthma medications. Check with your doctor.

Other nutrients which may help relieve asthma include vitamin C, vitamin B_6, niacinamide, pantothenic acid, and vitamin B_{12}. In addition, many asthmatics have unrecognized food allergies. A nutrition-oriented health care practitioner can help you identify foods in your diet that might be provoking asthma.

Other Respiratory Diseases

In addition to its beneficial effect in asthma, magnesium may also have value in the treatment of other respiratory disorders. In lung diseases such as emphysema, chronic bronchitis, and conditions that restrict movement of the lung tissue or chest wall muscles, the respiratory muscles must work especially hard to maintain the flow of air into and out of the lungs. This increased work load may be difficult for individuals with chronic lung disease, because many become malnourished and debilitated as their disease progresses. Although chronic lung disease is probably complicated by a wide range of nutritional deficiencies, magnesium appears to be especially important. Magnesium is required not only for inhaling and exhaling, but also to prevent the smooth muscles of the bronchial passages from going into spasm and choking off the air supply. To further complicate their tendency to become malnourished, patients with chronic lung diseases are often prescribed magnesium-depleting drugs, such as diuretics (water pills), digoxin, theophylline, and other bronchodilators. As a result, many such individuals are at risk for serious magnesium deficiency, which could further exacerbate their lung disease.

Because magnesium deficiency appears to be very common in people with chronic lung disease and supplementation may contribute to the development of respiratory muscle strength,[70] magnesium supplementation, either orally or by injection, should be considered.

Migraine

Migraine headaches cause severe, disabling pain among millions of Americans. Although numerous prescription drugs are available to prevent migraines and to treat acute attacks, none are completely successful. Factors that may promote migraines include cigarette smoking, caffeine ingestion, overconsumption of refined sugar, and use of oral contraceptives. Avoiding foods that contain a chemical called tyramine (such as aged cheese and certain wines), and identifying and avoiding allergenic foods (particularly wheat, citrus fruits, dairy products, eggs, yeast, and corn products) may help prevent migraines. An herb known as feverfew has also been reported to reduce the recurrence rate of migraines.

There is reason to believe that magnesium deficiency is one of the factors that promotes migraines and that supplementing with magnesium may reduce the number of attacks. For example, many situations known to provoke attacks of migraine (such as pregnancy, use of some diuretics, and ingestion of alcohol) are also known to deplete magnesium. Conversely, in certain areas of Africa and Japan where the dietary intake of magnesium is high, the incidence of migraine is among the lowest in the world.[71]

Drugs that are used to prevent or treat migraines usually have some of the same physiological effects as magnesium: (1) inhibiting blood vessel spasm, (2) inhibiting aggregation of platelets, (3) stabilizing cell membranes, or (4) interfering with the process of inflammation.[72] Drugs known as calcium channel blockers are currently popular for preventing migraines. It is noteworthy, therefore, that an article in the *American Heart Journal* referred to magnesium as nature's calcium channel blocker.[73]

Magnesium levels have been shown to be low during a migraine attack.[74,75] Thus, magnesium has been used with some success, both to prevent and to treat migraines.[76] One doctor has used magnesium to prevent migraines in more than 3,000 patients (almost all women), with a success rate of 80 percent. The usual dose was 200 mg per day.[77] Magnesium injections have also been reported to abort acute attacks of migraine.[78] I have found that a combination of magnesium, calcium, B vitamins, and vitamin C, given intravenously, can often relieve a migraine attack within one or two minutes.

Not all studies have found magnesium to be effective against migraines. Among one group of 50 patients who received 300 to 600 mg per day of magnesium for two months, none reported any improvement.[79] Further research is obviously needed to determine which types of individuals are most likely to benefit from magnesium. However, because of its safety and low cost, a trial of magnesium supplementation seems logical for most people who suffer migraines.

Fibromyalgia and Other Painful Conditions

Fibromyalgia is a common problem characterized by chronic pain and spasm in the muscles and surrounding tissue. The cause is unknown and treatment is only partially successful. Individuals with fibromyalgia also suffer frequently from fatigue and depression. Treatment includes antidepressants, muscle-relaxing drugs such as Valium, pain medications, antiinflammatory medications, physical therapy, and injections into "trigger points." However, despite the best that conventional medicine has to offer, millions of Americans continue to suffer from fibromyalgia.

Because of its beneficial effect on muscle spasm and fatigue, magnesium seems like a logical candidate for the treatment of fibromyalgia. In one study of more than 200 patients with chronic depression and/or pain, 75 percent had low levels of magnesium in their red blood cells or white blood cells. When magnesium was given intravenously to these patients, their symptoms improved rapidly. Muscle pain responded most often, but depression also improved.[80] These results were confirmed in a second study.[81]

Oral magnesium may also help relieve fibromyalgia, provided it is given in combination with another natural compound known as malic acid. In a recent report, 15 individuals with fibromyalgia received daily 300 to 600 mg of magnesium and 1,200 to 2,400 mg of malic acid. After four weeks, there was a significant improvement in muscle pain, which was even greater after eight weeks of treatment.[82]

Kidney Stones

Kidney stones are a common medical problem in the United States, affecting as many as 1 in 15 men and approximately half as many women. The incidence of kidney stones has nearly doubled in recent decades. People who have had one stone have a 50 percent chance of developing another one and, up to age 50, they have an 8 to 10 percent chance of a recurrence in any given year.

The majority of kidney stones contain calcium and oxalate. Magnesium inhibits the formation of calcium oxalate crystals and was suggested as early as the 17th century as a preventive for kidney stones. In a more recent study, 55 patients with recurrent kidney stones were given 500 mg per day of magnesium, in the form of magnesium hydroxide, for up to four years. During that time, the average annual recurrence rate fell by 90 percent; from 0.8 to 0.08 stones per person. As many as 85 percent of the patients receiving magnesium remained stone-free, compared to only 41 percent of a similar group of patients who did not receive magnesium.[83] Similar results were obtained in another study.[84] These studies, combined with the results of numerous animal experiments, indicate that magnesium has a powerful effect in preventing calcium oxalate kidney stones. Adding a small amount of vitamin B_6 may enhance the effect of magnesium.

Magnesium and Pregnancy

The development of a fetus into a healthy infant requires an adequate supply of all nutrients including magnesium. Since a pregnant woman is eating for two, it is important that she choose foods that contain enough vitamins, minerals, and high-quality protein. Unfortunately, many pregnant women do not make wise food choices.

A Wisconsin study found that 95 percent of pregnant women consumed less than 70 percent of the RDA for magnesium in their diet.[85] A number of complications of pregnancy may be due, at least in part, to suboptimal intake of magnesium. In animals, even a mild magnesium deficiency results in an increased number of fetal deaths and birth defects.

Several groups of researchers have studied the effect of magnesium supplementation in pregnant women. In one study, women who were given a magnesium supplement had a 29.5-percent lower risk of being hospitalized for pregnancy complications than those who received a placebo. The incidence of hemorrhages, incompetent cervix, and premature labor were all significantly reduced by administering magnesium. Compared to the placebo group, the magnesium group also had significantly fewer low-birth weight infants and infants with low Apgar score.[86]

Magnesium given intravenously is the standard treatment for a severe complication of pregnancy known as toxemia. Women with toxemia develop edema (fluid retention) and high blood pressure and are at risk for having seizures. Each year, hundreds of mothers and thousands of infants die as a direct result of toxemia. If intravenous magnesium can relieve the manifestations of toxemia after they have developed, then it is possible that ingesting enough magnesium throughout pregnancy would help prevent toxemia from occurring in the first place. In a double-blind study, pregnant women who took 465 mg per day of supplemental magnesium had a 41 percent lower incidence of toxemia than women who received only 100 mg per day.[87] Other research has shown that taking 10 mg per day of vitamin B_6 (a nutrient that often works in conjunction with magnesium)[88] reduced the incidence of toxemia by 61 percent.[89] Including enough protein in the diet is also important for preventing toxemia.

Premenstrual Syndrome

Premenstrual syndrome (PMS) is a symptom complex that affects as many as 70 to 90 percent of women of childbearing age. PMS symptoms usually begin several days to one week before menstruation, becoming more severe, and then stop abruptly as soon as the menstrual flow starts. Common complaints include emotional tension, depression, irritability, headaches, weight gain, fluid retention, swollen breasts, bloated abdomen, nausea, constipation, flare-ups of acne, and intense cravings for sweet or salty foods. In some women, these symptoms are only mild, but in others they are severe enough to interfere with normal activity for several days.

Engaging in regular aerobic exercise often improves the symptoms of PMS. Dietary modifications, such as avoiding refined sugar and moderating intake of salt, fat, and dairy products, is also beneficial in some cases. Nutritional supplements that have been shown to be effective for PMS include vitamin B_6, vitamin E and essential fatty acids, as well as magnesium. In difficult cases, natural progesterone has been used with success.

Because some of the symptoms of PMS are similar to those of magnesium deficiency, it is possible that magnesium deficiency is one of the causes of PMS.[90,91] To investigate that possibility, a group of Italian scientists studied the effect of magnesium supplementation on 32 women with PMS. Each woman received 360 mg per day of magnesium or a placebo for two months, in a double-blind trial. The supplements were taken daily from day 15 of the menstrual cycle until the onset of menstruation. Magnesium was significantly more effective than the placebo in relieving premenstrual mood changes.[92]

The evidence therefore suggests that magnesium supplementation is an important component of the treatment of PMS. Of course, as is often the case with individual nutrients, magnesium alone is unlikely to be as effective as a comprehensive program that includes diet, exercise, nutritional supplements, and possibly progesterone. One study found that blood magnesium levels were the same in women with and without PMS.[93] This contrasts with previously cited research and serves as a reminder that no single treatment is effective for everyone.

Menstrual Cramps

Guy E. Abraham, M.D. reported in 1978 that menstrual cramps can often be relieved by a combination of magnesium and vitamin B_6.[94] Abraham recommended 100 mg of each, every two hours as needed during menstruation, and four times a day throughout the rest of the cycle. Magnesium probably acts by helping relax the muscles of the uterus, resulting in relief of spasm and pain. Vitamin B_6 presumably increases the effectiveness of magnesium by increasing its transport into the cells. However, since large doses of vitamin B_6 have the potential to cause nerve damage, anyone wishing to try Dr. Abraham's treatment should consult a practitioner who is knowledgeable about nutrition.

In a few cases of severe menstrual cramps, my patients have obtained almost instant relief with an intravenous injection of magnesium, calcium, B complex vitamins, and vitamin C.[95]

Osteoporosis

Osteoporosis, or thinning of the bones, develops in about 30 percent of American women after the time of menopause. As many as 1.2 million women per year suffer a fracture as a direct result of osteoporosis. The medical costs associated with this epidemic are estimated to be $6.1 billion annually.

Most doctors focus on calcium supplements, estrogen replacement therapy, and exercise as a means of preventing osteoporosis. While this approach has value, it is only partially effective. Furthermore, because of the risk of cancer and other side effects, many women either cannot or will not take estrogen.

In my recent book *Preventing and Reversing Osteoporosis*,[96] I pointed out that many nutrients besides calcium (e.g., vitamin K, manganese, folic acid, vitamin B_6, boron, strontium, silicon, zinc, and copper) play a role in maintaining healthy bones. In addition, two other ovarian hormones, progesterone and DHEA (dehydroepiandrosterone), may be safer and more effective alternatives to estrogen. I suggested that a comprehensive approach including diet, nutrient supplementation, judicious hormone therapy, and avoidance of certain environmental pollutants might not only prevent osteoporosis, but actually reverse it.

One of the most important components of any osteoporosis program is magnesium. As much as 50 percent of all the magnesium in the body is in the bones. It should not be surprising, therefore, that studies have demonstrated a role for magnesium in the prevention and treatment of osteoporosis. Israeli scientists measured the magnesium status in 19 osteoporotic women. Sixteen of the 19 women were found to have significant magnesium deficiency, and to have abnormally large bone mineral crystals.[97]

This defect of bone crystal formation in magnesium-deficient women may be one of the factors that increases fracture risk. It is well known that not all women with osteoporosis develop fractures. Why are some women with thin bones protected, while others break their bones easily? It is likely that the quality of bone is as important as the quantity. Just as a thin crowbar can withstand more stress than a thin piece of chalk, so it is that well-formed bone crystals would provide more resistance and resiliency than improperly formed crystals. The amount of magnesium present is probably one of the factors determining how strong your bones will be.

Magnesium Builds Bones

In addition to its effect on bone quality, magnesium appears to play a role in maintaining or even increasing bone mass. In a study by Guy E. Abraham, M.D., 26 postmenopausal women were given a supplement containing 600 mg per day of magnesium. Bone density studies performed on the calcaneus bone (a bone in the foot) revealed an astounding 11 percent increase in bone mass after only eight to nine months of treatment.[98] The interpretation of this study is complicated by the fact that the women also received dietary advice, other nutritional supplements that may improve bone mass, and hormone replacement therapy. As a result, it is not possible to determine how much of the improvement was due to the magnesium. On the other hand, never before had anyone achieved anything close to an 11 percent increase in bone density in nine months. It is therefore possible that supplementing with a higher-than-normal amount of magnesium was a key factor in this surprising improvement.

That possibility was borne out by a recent report from Israel.[99]

Thirty-one postmenopausal women received magnesium supplements in doses of 250 to 750 mg per day for two years. Bone density increased between 1 and 8 percent in nearly three-quarters of the women and remained unchanged in most of the rest. In contrast, 17 women who did not take magnesium supplements had bone density losses of 1 to 3 percent. This study shows that magnesium supplementation alone can prevent or even reverse the loss of bone mass that typically occurs around the time of menopause. Since the improvement in the Israeli study was not as great as that observed by Dr. Abraham, it is clear that factors other than magnesium play a role in maintaining healthy bones. Nevertheless, magnesium appears to be extremely important for osteoporosis prevention, perhaps even more important than calcium supplementation.

Taking calcium supplements without additional magnesium can make an already existing magnesium deficiency worse.[100] It is therefore important to balance calcium with magnesium in your supplement program. There are many different opinions about the proper ratio of calcium to magnesium in the diet. The traditional ratio is two-to-one in favor of calcium (800 mg of calcium and 400 mg of magnesium). However, the study of Abraham suggests that the optimal ratio might be closer to one-to-one. Others have suggested that we should be consuming more magnesium than calcium. Although additional research is needed before we will know the optimal ratio of calcium to magnesium, I have been gradually moving away from the traditional two-to-one ratio. I often recommend 500 to 600 mg per day each of calcium and magnesium as part of an overall osteoporosis prevention program.

Magnesium and the Immune System

Magnesium is involved in a number of different ways in the functioning of the immune system.[101,102] It is necessary for the synthesis of antibodies, for the binding of certain immune cells to their targets, for the destruction of foreign invaders, and for some aspects of the inflammatory response. Magnesium deficiency increases the susceptibility of animals to chronic viral and fungal infections. Magnesium also appears to play a protective role in acute allergic reactions. Magnesium deficiency causes atrophy of the thymus, an important component of the immune system. Although all of the roles played by magnesium in immune function have not been worked out, it is clear that maintaining a healthy immune system requires adequate amounts of this important mineral.

HOW TO TAKE MAGNESIUM SUPPLEMENTS

The research I have cited provides a strong argument that you should supplement your diet with magnesium. However, there is a good deal of confusion about what type of magnesium is the most efficiently absorbed and utilized. I have found that magnesium aspartate may be especially effective for certain conditions, such as fatigue, muscle spasm, and cardiac arrhythmias. However, magnesium aspartate is relatively expensive and provides only a small amount of magnesium per tablet. Many other magnesium salts are commercially available, including gluconate, citrate, chloride, glycinate, amino acid chelate, carbonate, hydroxide, oxide, acetate, and lactate. Although claims have been made about the superiority of some forms of magnesium over others, these claims have not been backed up by research.

In one study, magnesium absorption was measured in a group of healthy female students. There was no difference in magnesium absorption from magnesium citrate/lactate, magnesium hydroxide, and magnesium chloride.[103] However, in another study, magnesium absorption from enterically coated magnesium chloride was 67 percent less than the absorption from magnesium acetate.[104] Apparently, enteric coating somehow impairs the absorption of magnesium. Recently, magnesium glycinate has been promoted as a preferred source of magnesium. However, in a study of nine patients with Crohn's disease, there was no difference in magnesium absorption from magnesium glycinate and magnesium oxide.[105] In a study in rats, six different magnesium salts were nearly equivalent as nutritional sources of magnesium.[106]

These studies suggest that it may not matter very much what type of magnesium you take. However, for individuals with poor absorption or certain chronic illnesses, some forms of magnesium may be more effective than others. Additional research is needed to clarify that issue.

There is also some disagreement about whether magnesium should be taken with meals or on an empty stomach. It is my opinion that magnesium should be taken with meals, both to enhance absorption and to reduce the chance of causing a stomachache.

SIDE EFFECTS AND PRECAUTIONS

In general, magnesium supplements are quite safe. However, excessive amounts may cause diarrhea. Some individuals are unusually sensitive to magnesium and develop diarrhea even with small doses. In those cases, magnesium may be better tolerated by taking even smaller amounts, three or four times a day with food. Individuals with chronic renal (kidney) failure may accumulate magnesium in their body if they take a supplement. Since excessive magnesium levels can be dangerous, people with renal failure should not take magnesium without medical supervision. If you are taking medication for diabetes, heart disease, or high blood pressure, you should also consult your doctor before taking magnesium.

INTERACTIONS WITH OTHER NUTRIENTS

There is some evidence that the effects of magnesium are enhanced by other nutrients, including vitamin B_6, vitamin E, thiamine, zinc, and essential fatty acids. Studies have shown that deficiencies of vitamin B_6 or vitamin E reduce tissue levels of magnesium.[107] Because nutrients work in the body as a team, magnesium therapy may work best when taken as part of a comprehensive multiple vitamin and mineral program.

REFERENCES AND NOTES

1 Schroeder HA. Losses of vitamins and trace minerals resulting from processing and preservation of foods. Am J Clin Nutr 1971;24:562–573.
2 Hall RH. The agri-business view of soil and life. J Holistic Med 1981;3:157–166.
3 Ebeling W. The relation of soil quality to the nutritional value of plant crops. J Appl Nutr 1981;33(1):19–34.
4 Morgan KJ, Stampley GL, Zabik ME, Fischer DR. Magnesium and calcium dietary intakes of the U.S. population. J Am Coll Nutr 1985;4:195–206.
5 White HS. Inorganic elements in weighed diets of girls and young women. J Am Diet Assoc 1969;55:38–43.
6 Singh A, Day BA, DeBolt JE, Trostmann UH, Bernier LL, et al. Magnesium, zinc, and copper status of US Navy SEAL trainees. Am J Clin Nutr 1989;49:695–700.
7 Gaby AR. B_6: The Natural Healer. Keats Publishing, New Canaan, CT, 1987.
8 Brenner S. Aluminium, hot water tanks, and neurobiology. Lancet 1989;1:781.
9 Fine BP, Barth A, Sheffet A, Lavenhar MA. Influence of magnesium on the intestinal absorption of lead. Environ Res 1976;12:224–227.
10 Singh NP, Thind IS, Vitale LF, Pawlow M. Intake of magnesium and toxicity of lead: an experimental model. Arch Environ Health 1979;34:168–173.
11 Raab W. Cardiotoxic effects of emotional, socioeconomic, and environmental stresses. In Bajusz E, Rona G (eds.). Myocardiology, vol I, 1970, pp. 707–713.
12 Henrotte JG. Type A behavior and magnesium metabolism. Magnesium 1986;5:201–210.
13 Henrotte JG. Type A behavior and magnesium metabolism. Magnesium 1986;5:201–210.
14 McGuire R. Type A stress a drain on magnesium. Med Tribune, May 15, 1985, p. 1.
15 Henrotte JG. Type A behavior and magnesium metabolism. Magnesium 1986;5:201–210.
16 Frustaci A, Caldarulo M, Schiavoni G, Bellocci F, Manzoli U, et al. Myocardial magnesium content, histology, and antiarrhythmic response to magnesium infusion. Lancet 1987;2:1019.
17 Bajusz E, Selye H. The chemical prevention of cardiac necroses following occlusion of coronary vessels. Can Med Assoc J 1960;82:212–213.
18 Chang C, Varghese PJ, Downey J, Bloom S. Magnesium deficiency and myocardial infarct size in the dog. J Am Coll Cardiol 1985;5:280–289.
19 Parsons RS, Butler T, Sellars EP. The treatment of coronary artery disease with parenteral magnesium sulphate. Med Proc 1959;5:487–498.
20 Malkiel-Shapiro B. Further observations on parenteral magnesium sulfate therapy in coronary heart disease: a clinical appraisal. S Afr Med J 1958;32:1211.

21 Rasmussen HS, Norregard P, Lindeneg O, McNair P, Backer V, et al. Intravenous magnesium in acute myocardial infarction. Lancet 1986;1:234–236.

22 Shechter M, Hod H, Marks N, Behar S, Kaplinsky E, et al. Beneficial effect of magnesium sulfate in acute myocardial infarction. Am J Cardiol 1990;66:271–274.

23 Woods KL, Fletcher S, Roffe C, Haider Y. Intravenous magnesium sulphate in suspected acute myocardial infarction: results of the second Leicester Intravenous Magnesium Intervention Trial (LIMIT-2). Lancet 1992;339:1553–1558.

24 Dyckner T, Wester PO. Ventricular extrasystoles and intracellular electrolytes before and after potassium and magnesium infusions in patients on diuretic treatment. Am Heart J 1979;97:12–18.

25 Seller RH. The role of magnesium in digitalis toxicity. Am Heart J 1971;82:551–556.

26 Tzivoni D, Keren A, Cohen AM, Loebel H, Zahavi I, et al. Magnesium therapy for torsades de pointes. Am J Cardiol 1984;53:528–530.

27 England MR, Gordon G, Salem M, Chernow B. Magnesium administration and dysrhythmias after cardiac surgery. A placebo-controlled, double-blind, randomized trial. JAMA 1992;268:2395–2402.

28 Vitale JJ, White PL, Nakamura M, Hegsted DM, Zamcheck N, et al. Interrelationships between experimental hypercholesterolemia, magnesium requirement and experimental atherosclerosis. J Exp Med 1957;106:757–767.

29 Ouchi Y, Tabata RE, Stergiopoulos K, Sato F, Hattori A, et al. Effect of dietary magnesium on development of atherosclerosis in cholesterol-fed rabbits. Arteriosclerosis 1990;10:732–737.

30 Davis WH, Leary WP, Reyes AJ, Olhaberry JV. Monotherapy with magnesium increases abnormally low high density lipoprotein cholesterol: a clinical assay. Curr Ther Res 1984;36:341–346.

31 Malkiel-Shapiro B. Further observations on parenteral magnesium sulfate therapy in coronary heart disease: a clinical appraisal. S Afr Med J 1958;32:1211–1215.

32 Browne SE. Intravenous magnesium sulphate in arterial disease. Practitioner 1969;202:562–564.

33 Browne SE. Intravenous magnesium sulphate in arterial disease. Practitioner 1969;202:562–564.

34 Neglen P, Qvarfordt P, Eklof B. Peroral magnesium hydroxide therapy and intermittent claudication. Vasa 1985; 14:285–288.

35 Wener J, Pintar K, Simon MA, Motola R, Friedman R, et al. The effects of prolonged hypomagnesemia on the cardiovascular system in young dogs. Am Heart J 1964;67:221–231.

36 Frustaci A, Caldarulo M, Schiavoni G, Bellocci F, Manzoli U, et al. Myocardial magnesium content, histology, and antiarrhythmic response to magnesium infusion. Lancet 1987;2:1019.

37 Resnick LM, Gupta RK, Laragh JH. Intracellular free magnesium in erythrocytes of essential hypertension: relation to blood pressure and serum divalent cations. Proc Natl Acad Sci 1984;81:6511–6515.

38 Motoyama T, Sano H, Fukuzaki H. Oral magnesium supplementation in patients with essential hypertension. Hypertension 1989;13:227–232.

39 Dyckner T, Wester PO. Effect of magnesium on blood pressure. Br Med J 1983;286:1847–1849.
40 Multiple Risk Factor Intervention Trial Research Group. Multiple risk factor intervention trial. Risk factor changes and mortality results. JAMA 1982;248: 1465–1477.
41 Henderson DG, Schierup J, Schodt T. Effect of magnesium supplementation on blood pressure and electrolyte concentrations in hypertensive patients receiving long term diuretic treatment. Br Med J 1986;293:664.
42 Cappuccio FP, Markandu ND, Beynon GW, Shore AC, Sampson B, et al. Lack of effect of oral magnesium on high blood pressure: a double blind study. Br Med J 1985;291:235–238.
43 Altura BT, Altura BM. The role of magnesium in etiology of strokes and cerebrovasospasm. Magnesium 1982;1:277–291.
44 Altura BT, Altura BM. The role of magnesium in etiology of strokes and cerebrovasospasm. Magnesium 1982;1:277–291.
45 Galland LD, Baker SM, McLellan RK. Magnesium deficiency in the pathogenesis of mitral valve prolapse. Magnesium 1986;5:165–174.
46 Coghlan HC. Magnesium in mitral valve prolapse syndrome. Magnesium Trace Elem 1990;9:319–320.
47 Fernandes JS, Pereira T, Carvalho J, Franca A, Andrade R, et al. Therapeutic effect of a magnesium salt in patients suffering from mitral valvular prolapse and latent tetany. Magnesium 1985;4:283–290.
48 Rosen H, Blumenthal A, Agersborg HPK. Effects of the potassium and magnesium salts of aspartic acid on metabolic exhaustion. J Pharm Sci 1962;51:592–593.
49 Cox IM, Campbell MJ, Dowson D. Red blood cell magnesium and chronic fatigue syndrome. Lancet 1991;337:757–760.
50 Clague JE, Edwards RHT, Jackson MJ. Intravenous magnesium loading in chronic fatigue syndrome. Lancet 1992;340:124–125.
51 Deulofeu R, Gascon J, Gimenez N, Corachan M. Magnesium and chronic fatigue syndrome. Lancet 1991;338:641.
52 For a description of intravenous vitamin and mineral therapy, see Gaby AR. *Preventing and Reversing Osteoporosis*, Prima Publishing, Rocklin, CA, 1994, pp. 277–279.
53 Brilla LR, Haley TF. Effect of magnesium supplementation on strength training in humans. J Am Coll Nutr 1992;11:326–329.
54 Brilla LR, Wenos DL. Perceived exertion to endurance exercise following magnesium supplementation. Magnesium Trace Elem 1990;9:319–320.
55 Gaby AR, Wright JV. Nutritional regulation of blood glucose. J Advancement Med 1991;4:57–71.
56 Hatwal A, Gujral AS, Bhatia RPS, Agrawal JK, Bajpai HS. Association of hypomagnesemia with diabetic retinopathy. Acta Ophthalmol 1989;67:714–716.
57 Ewald U, Gebbre-Medhin M, Tuvemo T. Hypomagnesemia in diabetic children. Acta Paediatr Scand 1983;72:367–371.
58 McNair P, Christiansen C, Madsbad S, Lauritzen E, Faber O, et al. Hypomagnesemia, a risk factor in diabetic retinopathy. Diabetes 1978;27:1075–1077.

59 Yajnik CS, Smith RF, Hockaday TDR, Ward NI. Fasting plasma magnesium concentrations and glucose disposal in diabetes. Br Med J 1984;288:1027–1028.

60 Paolisso G, Sgambato S, Gambardella A, Pizza G, Tesauro P, et al. Daily magnesium supplements improve glucose handling in elderly subjects. Am J Clin Nutr 1992;55:1161–1167.

61 Stebbing JB, Turner MO, Franz KB. Reactive hypoglycemia and magnesium. Magnesium Bulletin 1982;2:131–134.

62 Rayssiguier Y. Hypomagnesemia resulting from adrenaline infusion in ewes: its relation to lipolysis. Horm Metab Res 1977;9:309–314.

63 Phillips PJ, Vedig AE, Jones PL, Chapman MG, Collins M, et al. Metabolic and cardiovascular side effects of the ß2-adrenoceptor agonists salbutamol and rimiterol. Br J Clin Pharmacol 1980;9:483–491.

64 Durlach J. Magnesium and allergy: experimental and clinical relationships between magnesium and hypersensitivity. Rev Franc Allergol 1975;15:133–146.

65 Haury VG. Blood serum magnesium in bronchial asthma and its treatment by the administration of magnesium sulfate. J Lab Clin Med 1940;26:340–344.

66 Haury VG. Blood serum magnesium in bronchial asthma and its treatment by the administration of magnesium sulfate. J Lab Clin Med 1940;26:340–344.

67 Okayama H, Aikawa T, Okayama M, Sasaki H, Mue S, et al. Bronchodilating effect of intravenous magnesium sulfate in bronchial asthma. JAMA 1987;257:1076–1078.

68 Skobeloff EM, Spivey WH, McNamara RM, Greenspan L. Intravenous magnesium sulfate for the treatment of acute asthma in the emergency department. JAMA 1989;262:1210–1213.

69 For a description of intravenous vitamin and mineral therapy, see Gaby AR. *Preventing and Reversing Osteoporosis*, Prima Publishing, Rocklin, CA, 1994, pp. 277–279.

70 Molloy DW. Hypomagnesemia and respiratory-muscle weakness in the elderly. Geriatr Med Today 1987;6(2):53–61.

71 Altura BM. Calcium antagonist properties of magnesium: implications for anti-migraine actions. Magnesium 1985;4:169–175.

72 Altura BM. Calcium antagonist properties of magnesium: implications for anti-migraine actions. Magnesium 1985;4:169–175.

73 Iseri LT, French JH. Magnesium: nature's physiologic calcium blocker. Am Heart J 1984;108:188–193.

74 Baker B. New research approach helps clarify magnesium/migraine link. Family Pract News, August 15, 1993, p. 16.

75 Ramadan NM, Halvorson H, Vande-Linde A, Levine SR, Helpern JA, et al. Low brain magnesium in migraine. Headache 1989;29:590–593.

76 Faccinetti F, Sances G, Borella P, Gonazzani AR, Nappi G. Magnesium prophylaxis of menstrual migraine: effects on intracellular magnesium. Headache 1991;31:298–304.

77 Weaver K. Magnesium and migraine. Headache 1990;30:168.

78 Swanson DR. Migraine and magnesium: eleven neglected connections. Perspect Biol Med 1988;31:526–557.

79 Baker B. New research approach helps clarify magnesium/migraine link. Family Pract News, August 15, 1993, p. 16.

80 Shealy CN, Cady RK, Veehoff D, Burnetti M, Houston R, et al. Magnesium deficiency in depression and chronic pain. Magnesium Trace Elem 1990;9:333.

81 Reed JC. Magnesium therapy in musculoskeletal pain syndromes— retrospective review of clinical results. Magnesium Trace Elem 1990;9:330.

82 Abraham GE, Flechas JD. Management of fibromyalgia: rationale for the use of magnesium and malic acid. J Nutr Med 1991;3:49–59.

83 Johansson G, et al. Effects of magnesium hydroxide in renal stone disease. J Am Coll Nutr 1982;1:179–185.

84 Prien EL Sr, Gershoff SN. Magnesium oxide-pyridoxine therapy for recurrent calcium oxalate calculi. J Urol 1974;112:509–512.

85 McGuire R. Lack of magnesium in pregnancy eyed. Med Tribune April 17, 1985, p. 10.

86 Spatling L, Spatling G. Magnesium supplementation in pregnancy. A double blind study. Br J Obstet Gynaecol 1988;95:120–125.

87 Sibai BM, Villar MA, Bray E. Magnesium supplementation during pregnancy: a double-blind randomized controlled clinical trial. Am J Obstet Gynecol 1989:161:115–119.

88 Gaby AR. B_6: The Natural Healer. Keats Publishing, New Canaan, CT, 1987.

89 Wachstein M, Graffeo LW. Influence of vitamin B_6 on the incidence of pre-eclampsia. Obstet Gynecol 1956;8:177–180.

90 Abraham GE, Lubran MM. Serum and red cell magnesium levels in patients with premenstrual tension. Am J Clin Nutr 1981;34:2364–2366.

91 Sherwood RA, Rocks BF, Stewart A, Saxton RS. Magnesium and the premenstrual syndrome. Ann Clin Biochem 1986;23:667–670.

92 Facchinetti F, Borella P, Sances G, Fioroni L, Nappi RE, et al. Oral magnesium successfully relieves premenstrual mood changes. Obstet Gynecol 1991; 78:177–181.

93 Hagen I, Nesheim B-I, Tuntland T. No effect of vitamin B_6 against premenstrual tension. Acta Obstet Gynecol Scand 1985;64:667–670.

94 Abraham GE. Primary dysmenorrhea. Clin Obstet Gynecol 1978; 21(1):139–145.

95 For a description of intravenous vitamin and mineral therapy, see Gaby AR. Preventing and Reversing Osteoporosis, Prima Publishing, Rocklin, CA, 1994, pp. 277–279.

96 Gaby AR. Preventing and Reversing Osteoporosis, Prima Publishing, Rocklin, CA, 1994

97 Cohen L, Kitzes R. Infrared spectroscopy and magnesium content of bone mineral in osteoporotic women. Isr J Med Sci 1981;17:1123–1125.

98 Abraham GE, Grewal H. A total dietary program emphasizing magnesium instead of calcium. Effect on the mineral density of calcaneous bone in post-menopausal women on hormonal therapy. J Reprod Med 1990;35:503–507.

99 Vikhanski L. Magnesium may slow bone loss. Med Tribune, July 22, 1993, p. 9.

100 Smith KT, Luhrsen KR. Trace mineral interactions during elevated calcium consumption. Fed Proc 1986;45:374.

101 Galland L. Magnesium and immune function: an overview. Magnesium 1988;7:290–299.

102 Larvor P. Magnesium, humoral immunity, and allergy. In *Magnesium in Health and Disease*, Spectrum Publ. Inc., pp. 201–224.

103 Bohmer T, Roseth A, Holm H, Weberg-Teigen S, Wahl L. Bioavailability of oral magnesium supplementation in female students evaluated from elimination of magnesium in 24-hour urine. Magnesium Trace Elem 1990;9:272–278.

104 Fine KD, Santa Ana CA, Porter JL, Fordtran JS. Intestinal absorption of magnesium from food and supplements. J Clin Invest 1991;88:396–402.

105 Schuette S, Lashner B, Hartmann S, Du L, Janghorbani M. Bioavailability of Mg glycinate versus MgO in Crohn's disease patients with ileal resection. Magnesium Trace Elem 1990;9:332.

106 Cook DA. Availability of magnesium: balance studies in rats with various inorganic magnesium salts. J Nutr 1973;103:1365–1370.

107 Anonymous. Probe nutrient roles in heart diseases, cancer, and ileitis. Hosp Pract 1983(January):153.

Good Health Guides for Areas of Special Interest

MINERALS AND ACCESSORY NUTRIENTS

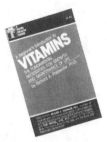

☐ A Beginner's Introduction to Trace Minerals	$2.00
Erwin DiCyan, Ph.D.	362-9
☐ Choline, Lecithin, Inositol	$2.25
Jeffrey Bland, Ph.D.	277-0
☐ Chromium Picolinate	$2.95
Richard A. Passwater, Ph.D.	588-5
☐ Coenzyme Q-10	$2.50
William H. Lee, R.Ph., Ph.D.	427-7
☐ Glandular Extracts	$3.50
Michael Murray, N.D.	611-3
☐ GTF Chromium	$2.25
Richard A. Passwater, Ph.D.	272-X
☐ Lysine, Tryptophan and Other Amino Acids	$2.25
Robert Garrison, Jr., R.Ph., M.A.	268-1
☐ Magnesium	$3.50
Alan L. Gaby, M.D.	602-4
☐ The New Superantioxidant— Plus	$2.95
Richard A. Passwater, Ph.D.	589-3
☐ Octacosanol, Carnitine	$2.25
Jeffrey Bland, Ph.D.	316-5
☐ Orotates and Other Mineral Transporters	$1.95
William H. Lee, R.Ph., Ph.D.	337-8
☐ The Picolinates	$1.95
Gary Evans, Ph.D.	511-5
☐ Selenium Update	$1.95
Richard A. Passwater, Ph.D.	393-9

MARVEL VITAMINS

☐ The Antioxidants	$2.50
Richard A. Passwater, Ph.D.	404-8
☐ A Beginner's Introduction to Vitamins	$2.50
Richard A. Passwater, Ph.D.	338-6
☐ Beta-Carotene	$2.50
Richard A. Passwater, Ph.D.	363-7
☐ Bioflavonoids	$2.50
Jeffrey Bland, Ph.D.	330-0
☐ Getting the Most Out of Your Vitamins and Minerals	$3.50
Jack Challem	605-9
☐ Vitamin B3 (Niacin) Updated	$2.25
Abram Hoffer, M.D., Ph.D.	513-5
☐ Vitamin C Updated	$1.95
Jack Challem	285-1
☐ Vitamin E Updated	$1.45
Len Mervyn, Ph.D.	274-6
☐ The Vitamin Robbers	$2.25
Earl Mindell, R.Ph., Ph.D. and William H. Lee, R. Ph., Ph.D	275-4

HOMEOPATHY AND ALTERNATE THERAPIES

☐ A Beginner's Introduction to Ayurvedic Medicine	$3.00
Vivek Shanbhag, M.D.(Ayur-Veda)	604-0
☐ A Beginner's Introduction to Homeopathy	$2.50
Trevor Cook, M.D.	394-7
☐ Lifetime Wellness	$1.95
Joan A. Friedrich, Ph.D.	477-3
☐ The Rinse Formula	$1.95
Jacobus Rinse, Ph.D.	465-X
☐ The Traditional Flower Remedies of Dr. Edward Bach	$2.25
Leslie J. Kaslof	463-3

SPECIFIC HEALTH PROBLEMS

☐ Candida Albicans Ray Wunderlich, Jr., M.D.	$2.50 364-5
☐ Chemical Sensitivity Sherry Rogers, M.D.	$3.50 634-2
☐ The Disease of Aging Hans Kugler, Ph.D.	$2.25 366-1
☐ Gluten Intolerance Beatrice Trum Hunter	$2.50 435-8
☐ How to Cope with Menstrual Problems Nikki Goldbeck	$2.25 300-9
☐ Hypoglycemia Marilyn Light	$2.25 302-5
☐ Lyme Disease Ronald L. Hoffman, M.D.	$3.50 617-2
☐ A Nutritional Guide for the Problem Drinker Ruth M. Guenther, Ph.D.	$1.95 295-9

BENEFICIAL OILS AND NATURAL NUTRIENTS

☐ Brewer's Yeast, Wheat Germ, Lecithin Beatrice Trum Hunter	$1.95 278-9
☐ EPA—Marine Lipids Richard A. Passwater, Ph.D.	$1.95 321-1
☐ Evening Primrose Oil Richard A. Passwater, Ph.D.	$2.50 263-0
☐ Fish Oils Update Richard A. Passwater, Ph.D.	$1.95 432-3
☐ Flaxseed (Linseed) Oil and the Power of Omega-3 Ingeborg Johnson, CH and James R. Johnson, Ph.D.	$2.50 505-2
☐ The Friendly Bacteria William H. Lee, R.Ph., Ph.D.	$2.50 494-9
☐ Grain Power Beatrice Trum Hunter	$3.50 647-4
☐ Propolis: Nature's Energizer Carlson Wade	$2.25 329-7
☐ Therapeutic Uses of Vegetable Juices Dr. Hugo Brandenberger	$3.50 578-8
☐ Tofu, Tempeh, Miso and Other Soyfoods Richard Leviton	$2.50 284-3